D0008342

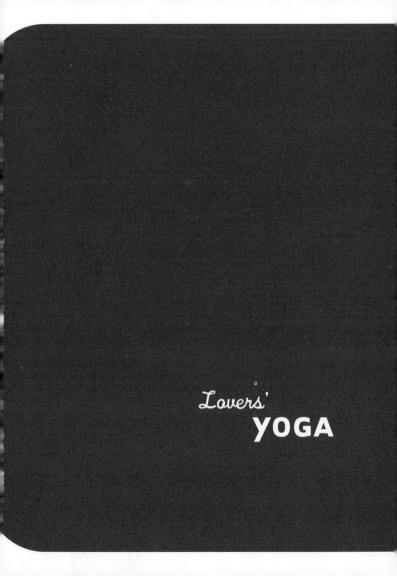

*Lovers'*
**YOGA**

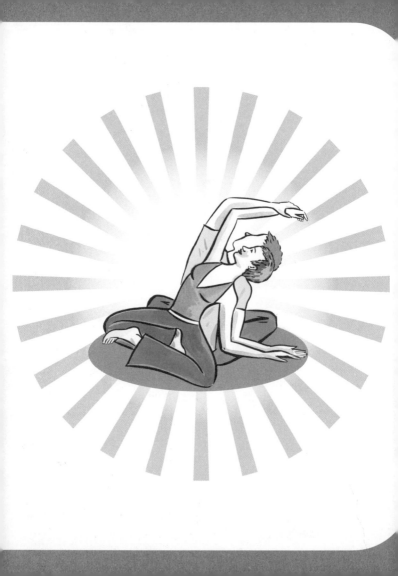

*Lovers'*
# YOGA

**soothing stretches** for two

By **Darrin Zeer**

Illustrations by **Thorina Rose**

CHRONICLE BOOKS
SAN FRANCISCO

Text Copyright © 2006 by Darrin Zeer.
Illustrations copyright © 2006 by Thorina Rose.

Library of Congress Cataloging-in-Publication Data:
Zeer, Darrin.
    Lovers' yoga : soothing stretches for two / by Darrin Zeer.
            p. cm.
    1. Hatha yoga. 2. Exercise for couples. 3. Stretching
exercises. I. Title.
    RA781.7.Z457 2005
    613.7'046—dc22
                                    2004030928
ISBN: 0-8118-4730-6

Manufactured in China

Designed by **Tim Belonax**

Distributed in Canada by Raincoast Books
9050 Shaughnessy Street
Vancouver, British Columbia V6P 6E5

10 9 8 7 6 5 4 3 2 1

Chronicle Books LLC
85 Second Street
San Francisco, California 94105

www.chroniclebooks.com

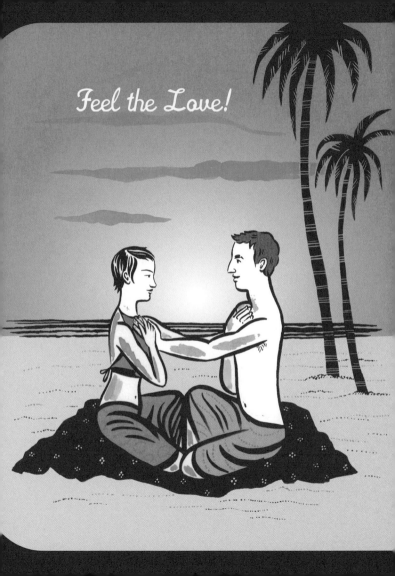

# contents

# Introduction

Welcome to *Lovers' Yoga*!

Our lives are so busy and stressful that we forget to take time out to simply relax. Quality time with your lover is often the first thing that is neglected. Like anything else in life, your relationship needs care and attention to grow.

Yoga is an incredibly rewarding way to spend time with your loved one. It's an age-old path to inner peace and wisdom that originated in India over five thousand years ago. It is revered as a way to relax the body, open the mind, and stay healthy. When you stretch with your partner, your bodies melt each other's tightness and tension. Simply by staying present, moment by moment, breathing in unison, a loving connection blossoms.

Whether your relationship is new or old, and whether you have a few minutes or a few hours, *Lovers' Yoga* will renew your connection and reinvigorate your life.

Organized into five chapters—Playful, Powerful, Peaceful, Patient, and Passionate Partner Yoga—this handy book features over fifty exercises that are easy and fun—whether you're a complete beginner or whether you've been practicing yoga for years. Feel free to experiment; just hang out in a particular pose that feels really good. Make sure to treat your partner well, because you can't do these stretches alone.

Once you get the hang of these stretches, start adding them into your daily life. Make a date to do the whole series on a Friday night. Try a pose or two after a long day to help you both decompress, or perform a calming stretch in the morning while you are waiting for the coffee to brew. Whether you are looking for romance or stress relief, you'll find the right pose in this book.

Feel free to do one stretch, a whole chapter sequence, or the entire book from beginning to end in one session. The exercises build on one another, so if you have the time, try the whole series. If you have a specific need, turn to the "Quickie Help Guide" on page 7.

And remember, first and foremost, take care of yourself and your partner!

## *Setting the Scene*

- If time permits, shower and put on fresh clothes. Choose a comfortable outfit that is easy to stretch in.

- Have some mints for fresh breath and drinking water handy.

- Turn off phones and try to limit other distractions.

- Music is helpful to set the mood. Keep a selection of your favorite CDs nearby.

- For a more romantic setting, light some candles.

- Keep pillows and a blanket handy; make sure you have enough room and remove any clutter.

## *Lover's Vows*

- I am grateful for this time with you.

- I will support you in the poses with care.

- I will listen and follow your every request.

- I will clearly communicate my needs.

- I will love and respect you.

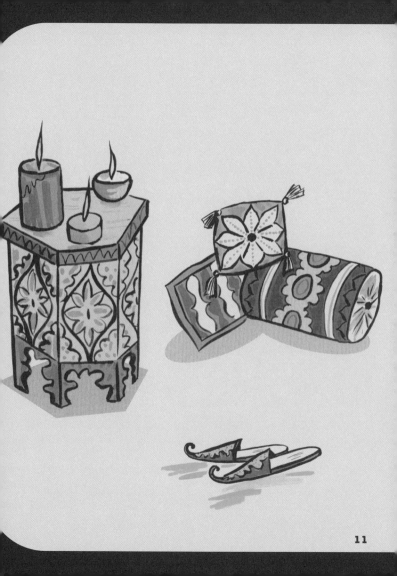

# part 1

# Playful Partner Yoga
## Standing Face-to-Face

**Take the time to have fun and unwind!**

*Connect with your partner!*

*Find your balance!*

*Don't worry—be happy!*

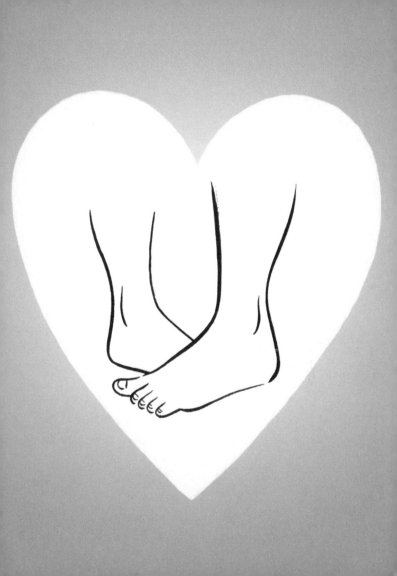

# *Partner Palm Play*

## *Flowing Hands*

- ¤ Stand face-to-face, about 2 feet apart.
- ¤ Gently rest your palms against your partner's palms.
- ¤ Feel the heat coming through his or her hands.
- ¤ Look into each other's eyes, relax, and breathe.
- ¤ Take 5 full breaths together.

## *Reach for the Sky*

- ¤ Press your palms firmly against your partner's palms.
- ¤ Together, reach your arms straight up.
- ¤ If you are shorter than your partner, grab on to his or her forearms.
- ¤ Rise onto your tiptoes and stretch up.

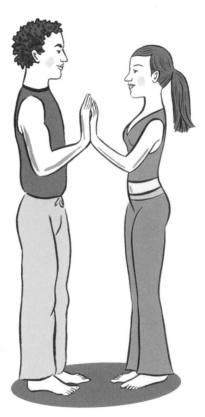

*Friendship needs no words.*
—Dag Hammarskjöld

## *Standing V for Victory*

- Stand face-to-face, about 1 foot apart.

- Firmly hold each other's arms and slowly lean back.

- To get a good stretch, make sure to stand tall and relax your arms and shoulders.

- Coach each other to relax and lean back farther.

- Take 5 long, deep breaths together.

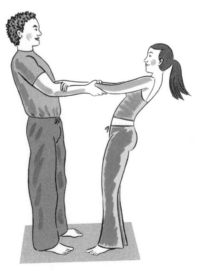

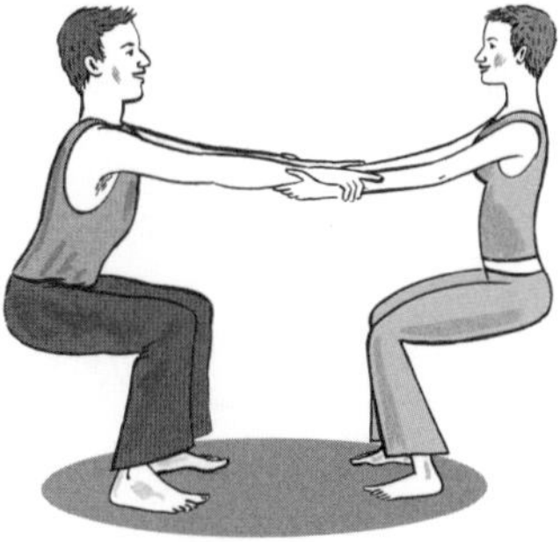

## Easy Chairs

- Stand face-to-face, about 3 feet apart, firmly holding each other's wrists.
- Bend your knees and slowly lower your buttocks onto invisible chairs. Smile and relax!
- Take 5 deep breaths and enjoy the strong leg workout.
- Support each other as you slowly rise back up.
- Repeat this stretch twice.

### *Advanced Moves:*

- Go down farther in your invisible-chair position, balancing together. Try not to let your buttocks touch the ground.
- Inhale slowly back up to standing position.
- Repeat this exercise 5 times, moving in unison.

# *Table for Two*

- ⌑ Stand face-to-face, 5 feet apart.

- ⌑ Keeping your legs straight, bend at the waist and drop forward so that your upper bodies form a tabletop.

- ⌑ Rest your hands on your partner's shoulders.

- ⌑ Relax into the stretch and breathe.

- ⌑ Try resting the tops of your heads against each other.

- ⌑ Take 5 deep breaths while you stretch.

- ⌑ Bend your knees and support each other on the way back up.

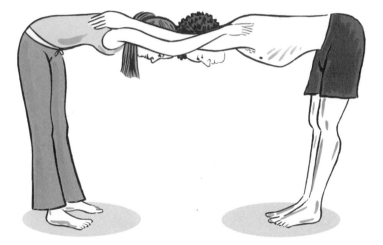

*Tension is who you think you should be. Relaxation is who you are.*
                                                    —*Chinese proverb*

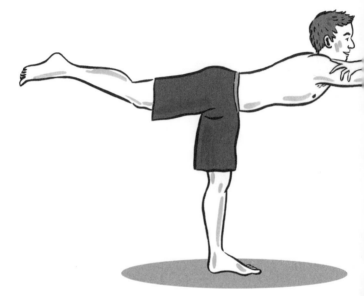

## T for Teamwork

⌑ Stand face-to-face, 1 foot apart, making sure the
space behind you is clear.

⌑ Take 3 long steps backward. With your left leg, take 1
big step toward each other.

⌑ Bend forward, putting your weight on your left leg,
and reach for each other's arms or shoulders.

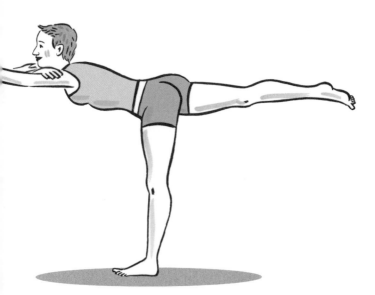

- ¤ Once you have a firm grip on your partner, kick your right leg back to make a "T" formation.

- ¤ Stand strong and hold tight, taking 5 deep breaths. Slowly release your hands and step your left foot back.

- ¤ Next, step forward with your right leg.

- ¤ Practice two sets for each leg.

# *Tree Together*

⌗ Stand side-by-side.

⌗ Lift your outside leg up
and place your foot on
your inside upper thigh.

⌗ If your foot slips, you
can hold it up with
your hand.

⌗ Wrap your inside arm
around your partner's waist
and hold tight for balance
and support.

⌗ Stand tall and feel
your head rise toward
the sky.

⌗ Breathe in unison and relax into the pose.

⌗ Take 5 deep breaths.

⌗ Switch sides with your partner and stretch the
other leg.

*Gratitude is not only the greatest of all
virtues, but the parent of all others.*

—Cicero

# Happy Hug

- Stand facing each other with toes touching.

- Hug!

- Relax deeply into your partner's embrace.

- Breathe 5 long, deep breaths in unison with your partner.

- Let stress and tension fall away.

## Easy Back Rub

- While still embracing, take turns massaging each other's back.

- Rest your head on your partner's chest or shoulder.

- Take turns rubbing each other's back between the shoulder blades and spine for 30 seconds.

## *Lovers' Meditation*
# LET-GO DANCE

◆◆◆ Listen to your favorite dance music.

◆◆◆ Move your hips to the rhythm of the beat.

◆◆◆ Let go and have some fun dancing.

◆◆◆ Stretch while you dance.

◆◆◆ Enjoy interacting with your partner.

◆◆◆ Take turns leading and following
each other.

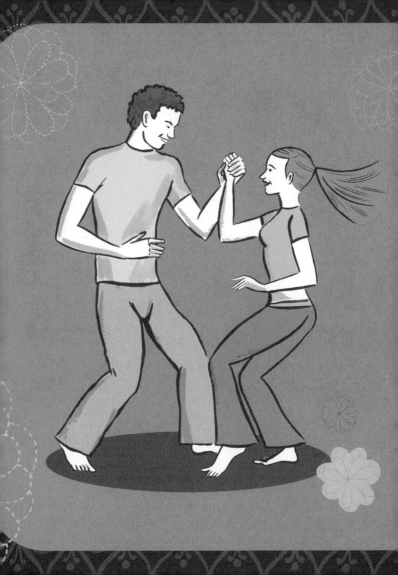

# part 2

# Powerful Partner Yoga
## Standing Back-to-Back

**Encourage each other to stand strong!**

*Stretch as a team!*

*Find your inner strength together.*

*Work out your body and your mind.*

**NOTE:** For this chapter, make sure you have space to move around and the floor is not cluttered or slippery. If you or your partner gets dizzy, be sure to sit down.

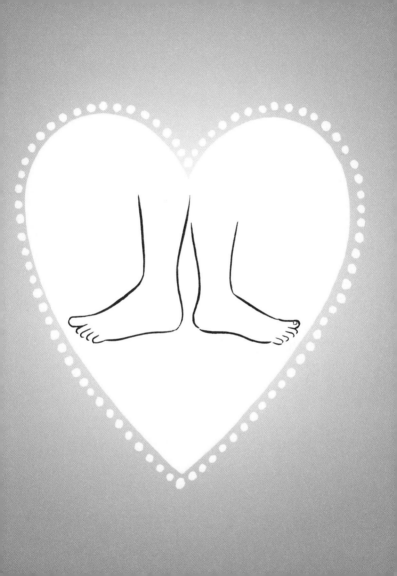

# Fanning the Flames of Love

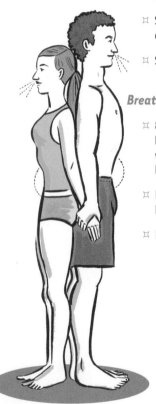

- ✡ Bodies Unite!

- ✡ Stand back-to-back. Reach down and hold your partner's hands.

- ✡ Stand tall and lean into each other.

### Breath of Fire

- ✡ Exhale rapidly through your nostrils by pumping your abdomen in. Don't worry about the inhale. It will happen naturally.

- ✡ Blow the breath from deep in your belly. Focus on deep, rapid exhalations.

- ✡ Do two sets of 15 exhales.

# Open-Your-Heart Stretch

- ⌑ Stand back-to-back, with your heels 1 or 2 feet apart.

- ⌑ Cross arms with your partner and decide who will receive the stretch first.

- ⌑ Raise your partner's arms to shoulder height and slowly stretch your partner's arms apart.

- ⌑ Remind your partner to relax his or her shoulders and chest. Take 5 deep breaths, and then switch positions.

# *Sweetheart Side Bends*

- Stand back-to-back, your hands touching your partner's hands.

- Bend your knees slightly and raise your arms up toward the sky together.

- Hold onto each other's hands or forearms, depending on the difference in your height.

- Press your backs together and slowly stretch to one side.

- Don't push it!

- Let your heads drop to the side.

- Hold for 5 deep breaths.

- When you're ready, raise your upper bodies up and slowly repeat the stretch to the other side.

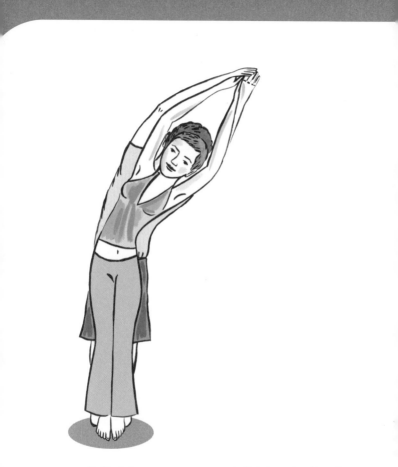

*Be kind, for everyone you meet is fighting a hard battle.*
—Plato

# *Trusting Triangle*

⌑ Stand back-to-back, about 1 foot away from each other.

⌑ Both raise your arms up to the sides, arms touching.

⌑ Together, take a big step in the same direction and turn your outer foot straight.

⌑ Bending at the waist, together tip your shoulders down toward the outer foot.

⌑ Lower your arms down and grab onto each other's leg.

⌑ Both reach your top arms up to the sky.

⌑ Touch your arms together to help each other balance.

⌑ Take 5 deep breaths together.

⌑ For support, let your bodies touch while you stretch.

⌑ Slowly rise up and repeat the stretch to the right.

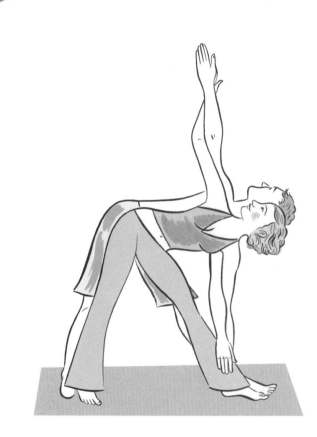

*Love is like the truth; sometimes it prevails, and sometimes it hurts.*
—*Victor M. Garcia Jr.*

# *Warriors of Love*

⊐ One partner stands about 1 foot behind the other.

⊐ Together, raise your arms out to the sides.

⊐ Both step about 3 to 4 feet to the left.

⊐ Turn the left feet straight out to the side.

⊐ Bend your left knees as far as is comfortable, making sure that the knee does not extend past the ankle.

⊐ Let your left arms point down to the ground.

⊐ The partner in front raises his or her right arm toward the sky.

⊐ The partner in back hugs the partner in front with his or her right arm.

⊐ Take 5 deep breaths together, then rise up and stretch to the right.

⊐ Do one set standing in front of and one set standing behind your partner.

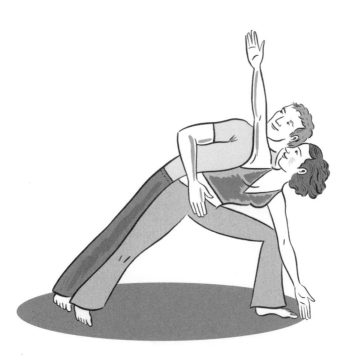

*Sorrow shared is halved, and joy shared is doubled.*
*—American Indian saying*

# Downward-Dog Duo

*Partner 1*

- ⌘ Firmly plant your hands and feet on the floor.

- ⌘ Separate your hands shoulder-width apart and your feet hip-width apart.

- ⌘ Slowly raise your hips to place your body in a "V" position.

- ⌘ Push back with your hands and stretch your heels toward the floor.

*Partner 2*

- ⌘ Stand facing your partner in front of his or her head, in between his or her hands.

- ⌘ Press your hands onto your partner's lower back and hold.

- ⌘ Gently massage up and down your partner's spine.

- ⌘ Take 5 deep breaths together and then switch positions.

*Advanced moves* (pictured below):

- ☐ Partner 1: Remains in the downward-dog position with Partner 2 standing away in front of his or her head.

- ☐ Partner 2: Slowly drape yourself face up over your partner's back into a backbend.

- ☐ Make sure your weight is not too heavy for your partner.

- ☐ Stretch your arms overhead to increase the stretch.

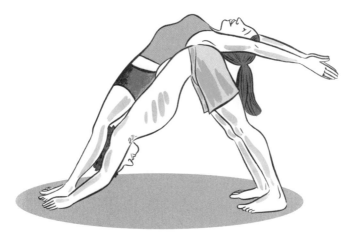

*Do not use a hatchet to remove a fly from a friend's forehead.*
—Chinese Proverb

# *Buddy Back Lift*

    ¤ Stand back-to-back and interlock elbows with
      your partner.

    ¤ Choose which partner gets stretched first.

*Partner 1*
    ¤ Make sure your buttocks are lower than your
      partner's by bending your knees.

    ¤ Get into a stable, balanced position.

    ¤ Slowly lean forward and lift your partner onto your back.

    ¤ Your partner's feet can lift slightly off the ground.

*Partner 2*
    ¤ Tell your partner how the stretch feels.

    ¤ Breathe, relax your body, and let your head rest back.

    ¤ Switch positions and repeat.

**Note:** This stretch is intense! If you are smaller than your
partner, you may not be able to lift him or her.

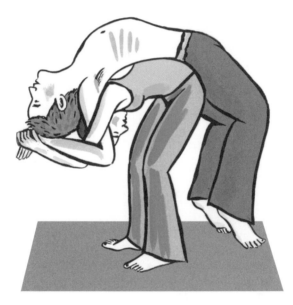

*Friends share all things.*
—*Pythagoras*

# Upside-Down Smile

- ⌑ Stand back-to-back, about 2 feet apart and separate your legs by about 3 feet.

- ⌑ Drop your upper bodies down like rag dolls, with arms hanging.

- ⌑ Look at your partner. Smile. Make funny faces.

- ⌑ If you can, grab onto your partner's arms or legs and pull yourself deeper into the stretch.

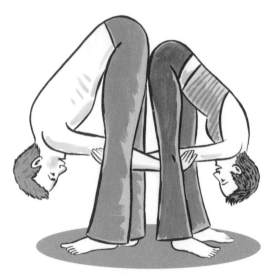

# *Powering-Down Pose*

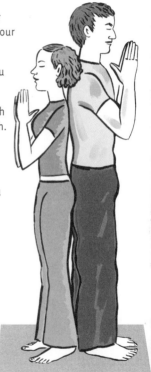

◻ Stand back-to-back.

◻ Hold your hands in the prayer position by your heart, with your eyes closed.

◻ Slowly inhale, counting as you breathe.

◻ Exhale, making the out-breath twice as long as the in-breath.

◻ Take 5 long, deep breaths together.

◻ Find balance and calm as you rest against your partner.

*Lovers' Meditation*

# SHARING CIRCLE

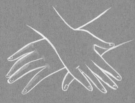

Sit comfortably face-to-face. Decide who will speak and who will listen.

*Instructions for the speaker:*

♦ Speak freely; say what you feel.

♦ Don't put pressure on yourself; what you say doesn't have to make sense.

♦ Talk about how you feel, avoiding negative or blaming comments about your partner.

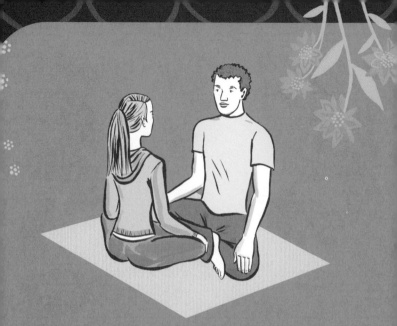

*Instructions for the listener:*

- Set a stopwatch for a particular time limit
  (2 minutes or more).

- Stay focused and caring while your partner shares;
  simply listen!

- Do not respond with any words or gestures.

- Switch roles and repeat exercise.

*part 3*

# Peaceful Partner Yoga
## *Sitting Back-to-Back*

**Effortlessly relax together!**

*Stay connected with your partner.*

*Let go of your stress and worries.*

*Melt into each other.*

**NOTE:** You can do this series on a large futon, thick mat, or padded carpet. Have pillows close by, to sit on and to use as props.

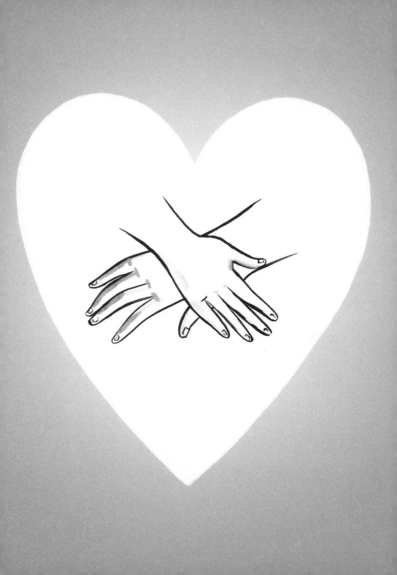

# Lean on Me

- Sit back-to-back, with your legs crossed or straight out in front.

- Rest your backs against each other and interlock arms, letting the backs of your heads touch each other.

- Bend together from the waist and make wide circles with your backs.

- Flow together in slow motion in both directions. Inhale to a count of 6 and exhale to a count of 6.

- Take 5 more of these breaths together and feel the deep relaxation.

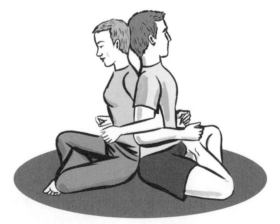

## *Seductive Side Bends*

⌑ Sit back-to-back, with legs crossed.

⌑ Drop your elbows down to one side and rest on your forearms.

⌑ Reach your other arms toward the sky.

⌑ Let your heads drop, and stretch to the side.

⌑ Hold for 5 deep breaths and then switch sides.

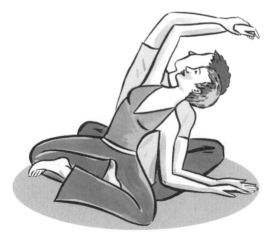

## *Tantric Twist*

⊐ Sit back-to-back, with legs crossed. Keep your lower backs as close together as possible.

⊐ Twist around to your left.

⊐ Place your left hand on your partner's right knee. Place your right hand on your own left knee.

⊐ Look behind you and relax your neck, pulling firmly on your partner's knee.

⊐ Take 5 deep breaths together.

⊐ Switch directions and repeat.

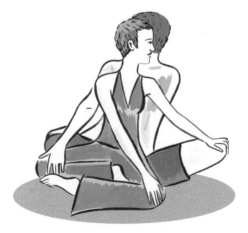

# Movin' on Up!

- ⌂ Squat back-to-back and interlock arms with your partner and lean against each other for balance.

- ⌂ On the inhale: Together, rise all the way up until you are both standing.

- ⌂ On the exhale: Slowly sit back down together.

- ⌂ Try going up and down 5 times slowly.

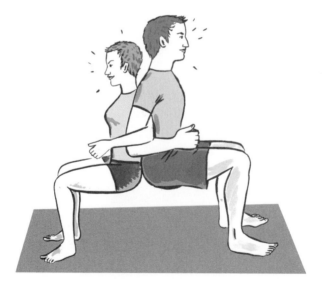

# *Blissful Butterflies*

- Sit back-to-back.

- Bring the soles of your own feet together.

- Relax!

- Let your knees slowly drop out to the sides and breathe into your groin and hip area.

- Press your legs down gently with your hands or elbows.

- Push your back against your partner's for leverage.

- You can also try reaching back and gently pushing down on your partner's knees.

- Relax your buttocks to go deeper into this stretch.

- Hold for 5 deep breaths.

- Make sure you release very slowly out of this stretch.

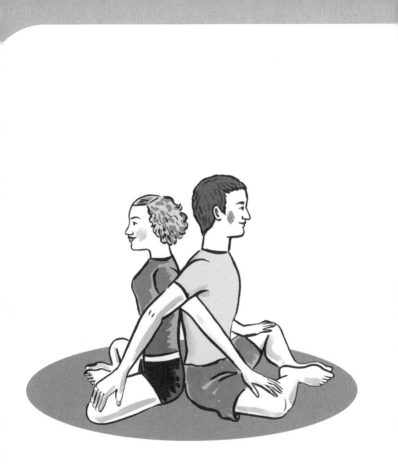

*You have no friends; you have no enemies; you have only teachers.*
*—Ancient saying*

# *Buddy Bends*

Sit back-to-back in preparation for a forward bend and backbend together.

*Partner 1*
- ⌑ Stretch your legs out in front of your body. It's OK if your knees are bent!

- ⌑ Drop your body into a forward bend, arms resting in front of you.

- ⌑ Get comfortable, breathe, and relax.

*Partner 2*
- ⌑ Cross your legs. Stretch back onto your partner's back, being careful to ask if the stretch is too intense.

- ⌑ Try crossing your arms and stretching them back and overhead.

- ⌑ Go slowly and relax into this stretch.

Take 5 deep breaths together. Be gentle; this is an intense pose for both partners. Release and switch directions.

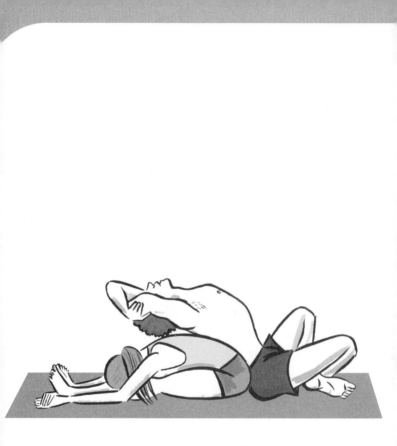

*Love truth, but pardon error.*
—*Voltaire*

## *Soothing Stretch Series*

### *Part 1:*

*Partner 1*

⌷ Lie face down, flat on the ground.

*Partner 2*

⌷ Squat onto your partner's buttocks, facing toward his or her head, making sure your weight is not too much for him or her.

⌷ Hold onto your partner's shoulders and slowly pull upward.

⌷ While in the stretch, your partner should tighten his or her buttocks to protect the lower back.

⌷ Hold him or her in the stretch for a count of 10, then release and rest. Repeat twice.

⌷ To end, give your partner a 30-second lower-back massage.

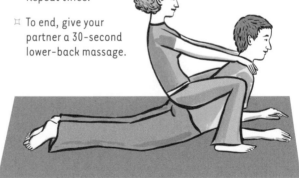

# Part 2:

*Partner 2*

- ⌘ Help your partner up from the ground.

- ⌘ Have your partner rest his or her upper body on the knees, arms in front of the body in the Child's Pose.

- ⌘ Kneel behind and face toward him or her.

- ⌘ Lie face down on top of your partner's back, with your legs spread apart. Ask if your weight is OK!

- ⌘ Take 5 deep breaths together and relax.

# Part 3:

Both partners lie flat on the floor, partner 2 on top of partner 1.

*Partner 2*

- ⌘ Make sure your weight is not too much for your partner.

- ⌘ Turn your heads in opposite directions and rest your arms at your sides.

- ⌘ Take 5 deep, relaxing breaths together, letting tension melt away.

# Part 3 *(continued):*

    ⌑ Next, partner 2 lies over partner 1's body at a
       right angle.

    ⌑ Roll your body over him or her like a steamroller.

    ⌑ Repeat from head to toe and back again a couple
       of times.

**Note:** Partners slowly rise up and switch roles. Repeat
      the three parts from beginning to end. Try Part 3
      whenever you or your partner needs quick
      stress relief.

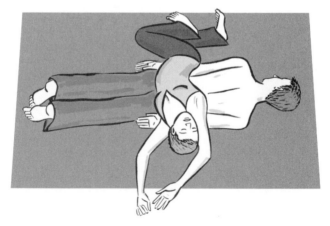

# *Melting into One Another*

- ⌑ Both partners lie down, facing each other, with the lighter partner resting on top of the heavier partner.

- ⌑ The bottom partner can wrap his or her arms around the top partner.

- ⌑ Breathe together in unison. Feel the deep relaxation.

*Variation* (pictured below):

- ⌑ Partners lie in opposite directions with only the sides of their heads touching.

- ⌑ With your heads snuggled together, check in with your partner and see how he or she is doing.

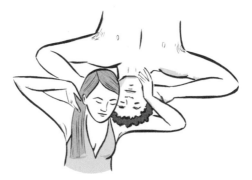

## *Lovers' Meditation*
# FINDING FORGIVENESS

Use this silent meditation as an opportunity to practice forgiveness in your relationship. Start by setting up a meditation space: dim the lights, limit distractions, and play some soft music. You can either lie or sit next to one another, but just focus on yourself for the first three parts. Close your eyes and spend at least 20 minutes on this silent meditation.

> Part 1: Calm yourself. Breathe and relax until you feel some peace of mind. Begin to focus your thoughts on your relationship.

> Part 2: Is there anything that you have done to your partner in the past that you feel bad about? Identify these interactions. Make a commitment to yourself to end the guilt or shame that you may be feeling.

> Part 3: Is there anything about your partner that you don't like? Focus on letting go of old judgments or resentments. Don't let the past get in the way!

> Part 4: To end this meditation, cuddle together with your partner. Just relax and hold each other with care.

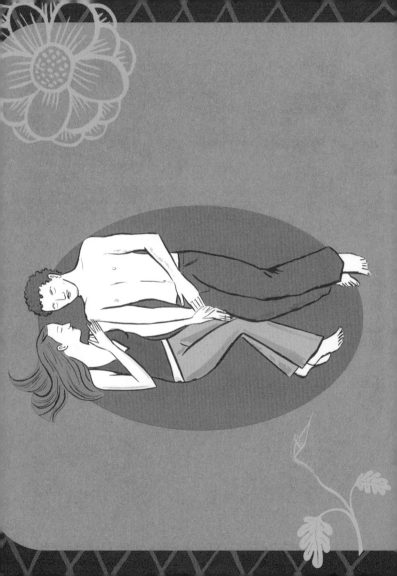

# Patient Partner Yoga
## *Sitting Face-to-Face*

**Be supportive and encouraging!**

*Always respect one another.*

*Communicate your needs.*

*Look deeply into each other's eyes.*

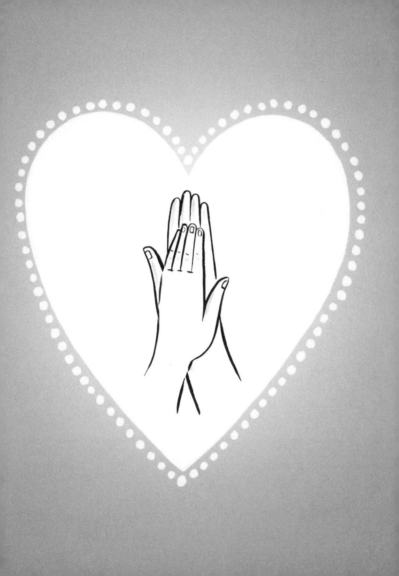

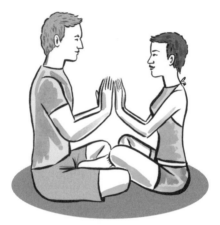

## *Tantric Dance*

- ⌕ Sit face-to-face, with legs crossed.

- ⌕ Look into each other's eyes, with your backs straight.

- ⌕ Bring the palms of your hands close together but not quite touching. Feel the heat and energy exchange between your hands.

- ⌕ Take 5 or more deep breaths in unison.

- ⌕ End this pose by touching your palms ever so gently together.

# Couple's Cat and Cow

- Sit face-to-face, with legs crossed and hands on each other's legs.

- Inhale while arching backward; let your chests rise as your heads drop back.

- Exhale, dropping your heads forward; let your shoulders slump.

- Breathe 5 inhales and 5 exhales together.

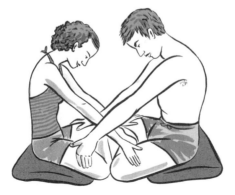

# Couple's Camel

⌑ Kneel face-to-face, about 1 foot apart.

⌑ Grasp your partner's arms firmly.

⌑ Both bend backward, stretching your chests to the sky and letting your heads drop back.

⌑ Both tighten your buttocks to protect your lower backs.

⌑ Communicate on how you can help each other balance.

⌑ Relax and enjoy this back stretch.

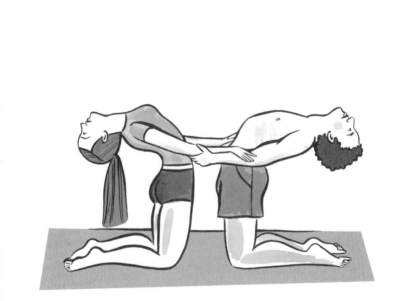

*The love we give away is the only love we keep.*
—Elbert Hubbard

# Flyin' High

Prepare for flight!

- Sit face-to-face, with knees bent and legs out in front of you.

- Press the balls of your feet against the balls of your partner's feet.

- Both partners grasp the other's hands firmly on the outside of their legs.

- Both partners press their feet together and slowly raise their legs.

- Smile and take 5 deep breaths together.

- Have fun balancing!

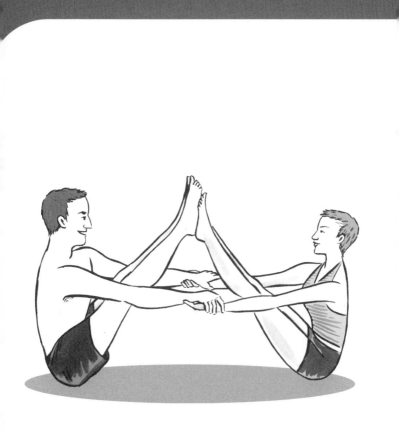

*Life is short. Be swift to forgive! Make haste to be kind.*
*—Henri F. Amiel*

## *Tug o' Love*

- ⌑ Sit face-to-face, legs stretched out in front of you, with the soles of your feet touching your partner's.

- ⌑ Reach forward and grab onto your partner's hands.

- ⌑ Take turns slowly stretching each other forward and back.

- ⌑ Hold each other in the stretch for 5 breaths.

- ⌑ End this stretch with an extended pull forward for each of you.

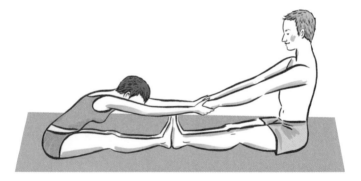

# *Rock the Boat*

⊐ Sit face-to-face, with your legs spread out wide.

⊐ Press the soles of your feet against your partner's
to create a diamond shape. Take hold of each other's
wrists.

⊐ One partner gently pulls the other partner forward.

⊐ The partner stretching back lets his or her chest rise
up and head drop back.

⊐ Imagine you are both rowing a boat. Take one breath
forward and one breath back.

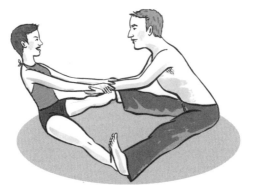

# *Sideways Smile Stretch*

⌑ Sit face-to-face, with your legs spread out wide, the soles of your feet touching your partner's.

⌑ Grasp your partner's left arm with your own.

⌑ Both reach your right arms overhead and stretch toward your left feet.

⌑ Pull on your partner's left arm to go farther into this stretch.

⌑ Drop your heads to the left and enjoy.

⌑ Be gentle, relax, and take 5 deep breaths.

⌑ Release and repeat this stretch on the right side.

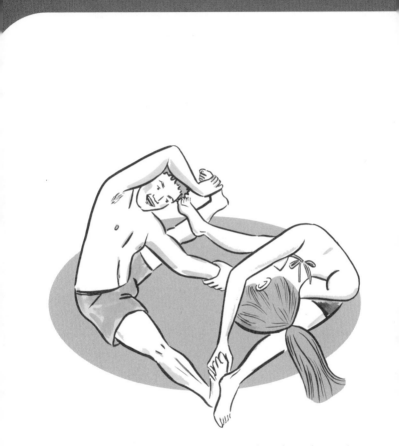

*Love me when I least deserve it,*
*because that's when I really need it.*
—Swedish proverb

# *"Heeling"* Massage

*Partner 1*

- ⌘ Have your partner sit up with his or her legs straight out in front.

- ⌘ Sit about 3 feet behind him or her, facing his or her back. Then, lie down and rest your feet on your partner's back.

- ⌘ Walk your heels up and down and rub the sore spots in between his or her spine and shoulder blades.

- ⌘ Rest your heels on top of his or her shoulders and push down. For extra leverage, raise your pelvis off the ground.

- ⌘ This is a heavenly way to give a back massage without lifting a finger.

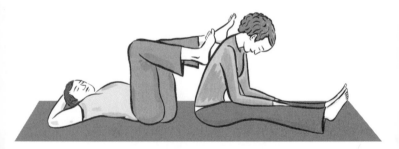

# *Heavenly Pose*

*Partner 1*

- Sit comfortably behind your partner.

- Place some pillows behind your back for support.

- Let your partner's body gently lie back on your chest.

- Help him or her to completely relax.

- Place one hand on the receiver's heart and one hand on his or her forehead.

- Breathe 10 or more times in unison.

- Rest deeply together.

- To end this pose, give your partner a tender scalp massage.

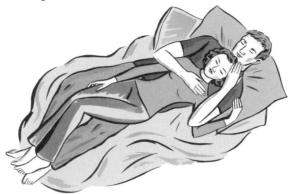

## Lovers' Meditation
# ACKNOWLEDGMENT CEREMONY

◆ Think about particular qualities you really like in your partner.

◆ Feel free to write down your thoughts.

◆ Take turns sharing your acknowledgments.

◆ Begin your sharing with the words "I love how you . . ." or "I loved it when you . . ."

◆ Let each other's kind words touch your hearts.

◆ Listen and be open.

◆ Thank your partner each time he or she shares.

◆ Hug each other once you are done; enjoy the intimacy and warm feelings.

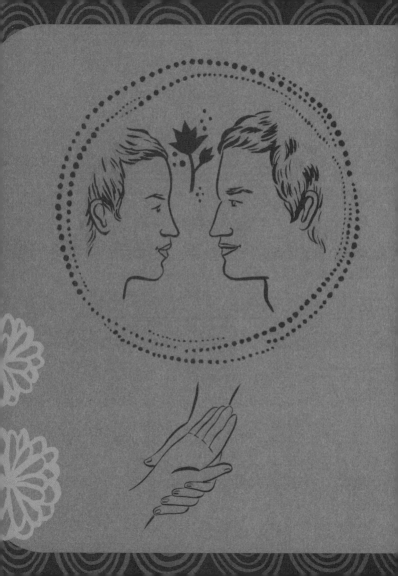

*part 5*

# Passionate Partner Yoga
## *Giving and Receiving*

. . . . . . . . . . . . . . . . . . . . . . . . . . . . . . .

**Connect and be intimate with each other!**

*Give your partner your full attention.*

*Surrender your body into the stretches.*

*Enjoy the powerful heart-opening experience.*

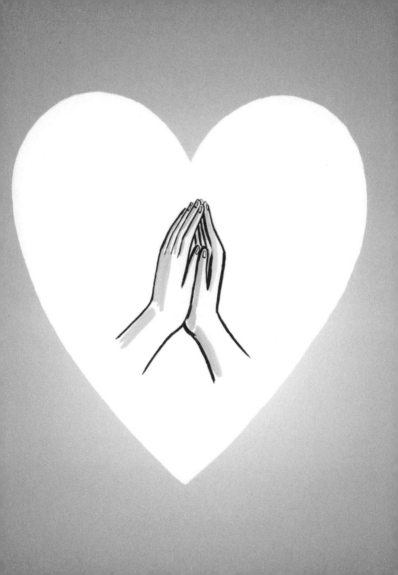

# Instructions for Partners

The giver in these stretches will take the receiver through the entire series, then you will switch roles. For maximum comfort, it's best to do these stretches on a large bed or futon.

## Instructions for receiving:

⌗ Trust the giver to take good care of your body. Tell the giver if you want to be stretched more or less.

⌗ Help the giver lift your body if your legs are too heavy for him or her.

⌗ Once in the stretch, let your entire body relax and take many long, deep breaths.

## Instructions for giving:

⌗ Move the receiver's body slowly and with care, especially as you take him or her out of each stretch.

⌗ Don't forget to ask the receiver if he or she is comfortable and wants to be stretched more or less.

⌗ For nurturing support, gently massage the receiver as he or she is being stretched.

⌗ Make sure your body is comfortably positioned as you give the stretches. Change your leg position from time to time to avoid becoming stiff and sore.

# *Loving Lap Hug*

- ⌨ Both partners sit down facing each other.

- ⌨ The receiver rests his or her legs on top of the giver's legs.

- ⌨ Sit close together and hug each other.

- ⌨ You both can loosely wrap your legs around each other.

- ⌨ The receiver rests his or her head on the giver's chest or shoulder.

- ⌨ Both partners close their eyes and take 5 or more deep breaths.

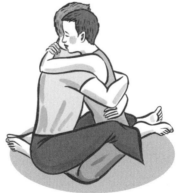

*Love takes off masks that we fear we cannot live without and know we cannot live within.*

—James Baldwin

## *Loving Support*

Both partners sit down facing each other.

*Giver:* Make sure the receiver's legs are resting on top of your legs.

⌗ Lower the receiver down so he or she lies flat on the floor.

⌗ Offer loving support by placing your hands on the receiver's belly or legs.

⌗ Remind the receiver to relax and breathe.

⌗ Take 5 or more deep breaths in unison.

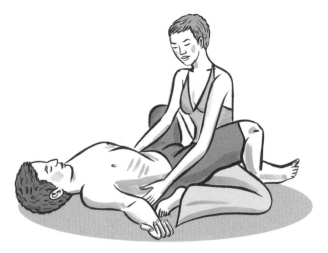

# Knee Circles

⊐ *Giver:* Sit kneeling or cross-legged.

⊐ Have the receiver lie on his or her back and rest the receiver's feet on your chest.

⊐ Take hold of the receiver's knees and rotate his or her legs in wide circles.

⊐ Go slowly and take 5 or more deep breaths together.

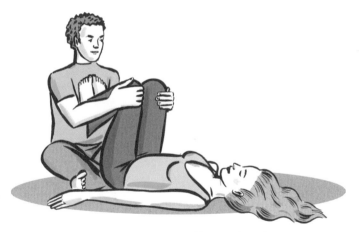

*Water and words are easy to pour,*
*but impossible to recover.*

—Chinese Proverb

# *Butterfly Opening*

- ✠ *Giver:* Sit with your legs crossed or straight.

- ✠ Have the receiver lie on his or her back.

- ✠ Rest the soles of the receiver's feet on your belly.

- ✠ Slowly let the receiver's knees drop in opposite directions.

- ✠ Use your legs as a support under his or her legs.

- ✠ Ask the receiver if he or she wants more or less of a stretch. To increase the stretch, press your elbows on his or her legs.

- ✠ Have the receiver take 10 or more deep breaths.

- ✠ Very slowly and gently raise the receiver's knees back together.

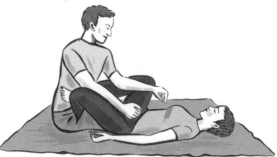

# Hip Bend

- *Giver:* Sit with your legs crossed or straight.

- Have the receiver lie on his or her back.

- Cross the receiver's left ankle in front of his or her right thigh.

- Bend the receiver's right leg and gently push it forward, asking how far he or she wants to be stretched.

- Have the receiver take 10 or more deep breaths.

- Slowly and gently release, then stretch the receiver's other leg.

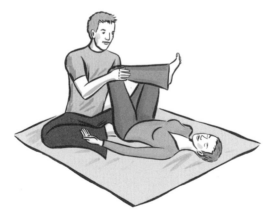

# Hip Twist

⊐ *Giver:* Sit with your legs crossed or straight.

⊐ Have the receiver lie on his or her back and inter-
lace his or her hands behind the head, with elbows
relaxed back.

⊐ Bend the receiver's legs and gently push the knees to
the chest.

⊐ Lower both of the receiver's knees slowly to his or her
left side.

⊐ Gently massage the receiver's hip and have the
receiver take 10 or more deep breaths.

⊐ Slowly lift his or her legs back up and repeat on the
other side.

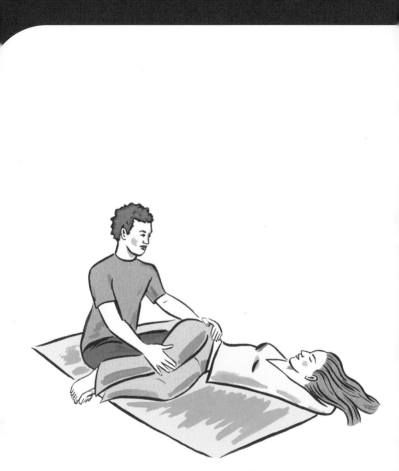

*I felt it shelter to speak to you.*
—Emily Dickinson

# *Uplifting Leg Stretch*

- *Giver:* Sit with your legs crossed or straight.

- Have the receiver lie on his or her back with the legs down, resting on top of your legs.

- Take hold of the receiver's right leg and lift it straight up.

- Place your left hand on the receiver's right heel and push forward.

- Brace the front of the receiver's right knee with your right hand.

- Make sure the receiver's right knee is held straight, and push his or her leg forward to increase the stretch.

- Have the receiver take five or more deep breathes.

- Slowly and gently release, then stretch the receiver's other leg.

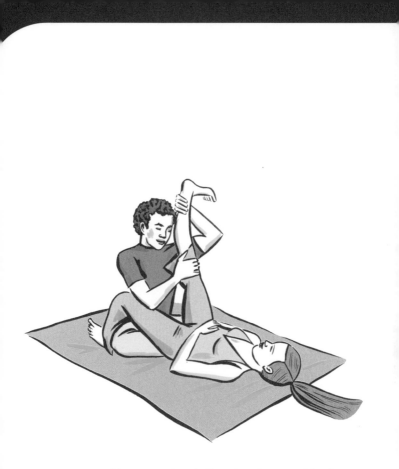

*A happy marriage is the union of two good forgivers.*
—*Socrates*

# *Romantic Roll*

- ⌑ *Giver:* Sit kneeling or cross-legged.

- ⌑ Take hold of the receiver's heels and slowly bend the legs at the knees and push his or her legs up to the chest.

- ⌑ Keep pushing until the receiver's lower back starts lifting off the ground.

- ⌑ Push the receiver's legs so that it looks like he or she is going to roll over.

- ⌑ Squeeze the soles of his or her feet for encouragement.

- ⌑ Ask the receiver how far he or she wants to stretch.

- ⌑ Have the receiver take 5 or more deep breaths.

*For a more intimate and intense stretch* (pictured opposite):

- ⌑ Slowly raise your body over the top of the receiver's legs.

- ⌑ Let your body weigh down on top of the receiver's bent legs.

- ⌑ Brace your arms on the ground to control the level of your weight.

- ⌑ Make sure the pressure is not too much for the receiver.

- ⌑ Take 10 or more deep breaths together.

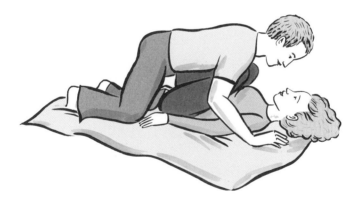

*A friend is a person with whom I may be sincere.*
*Before him I may think aloud.*

—Ralph Waldo Emerson

## Lovers' Meditation
# SPOONING SAVASANA

- ¤ The ultimate pose to melt into each other!

- ¤ Lie down, one partner behind the other.

- ¤ The partner in back can hug the partner in front.
  (Whoever needs the most nurturing should lie in front.)

- ¤ Breathe and relax, without any expectations.

- ¤ Your bodies will naturally connect together.

- ¤ Breathe in unison 10 or more times.

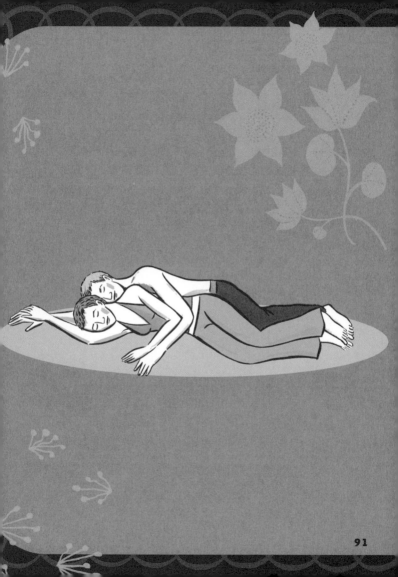

# *Lovers' Yoga in the Water*

If you have access to a large Jacuzzi or a heated pool, try a lovers' water-yoga session! Take turns being the giver and receiver. It's helpful to have a water flotation noodle to place underneath the receiver's knees. Ideally, the water should be 90° to 100°F and be 3 to 5 feet deep. Make sure neither of you overheats. Have drinking water close by.

## Head Snuggle

- *Giver:* Place some kind of a flotation device under the receiver's knees.

- Position yourself at the receiver's head and rest his or her head on your shoulder.

- Use both of your hands to massage the receiver's neck and back.

- To help loosen the receiver up, use your arms and rock his or her body from side to side. The water will do the work for you.

- End this by very gently holding your partner motionless.

## Caring Cradle

✠ *Giver:* Have the receiver lie back in the water and relax.

✠ Cradle the receiver in your arms, keeping his or her mouth and eyes above water.

✠ Gently hold the receiver's head with one arm and use your other arm to rock and massage the receiver's back.

✠ Go slowly and let the water do the work for you.

✠ Ask the receiver to keep his or her eyes closed and simply breathe and let go of control.

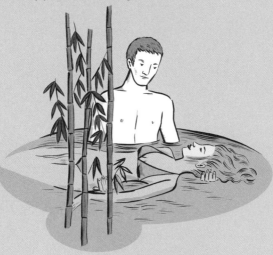

# The Happy Couple

Lovers' Yoga is a fun adventure—a journey into intimacy and relaxation with your partner.

The key to Lovers' Yoga is connecting with your partner. The poses are simply a doorway for both of you to step deeper into your relationship. By letting go of fears and tension, a peaceful intimacy will unfold. A tantric connection that will energize and relax both of you on all levels: body, mind, and spirit.

*Make this commitment here and now:* Care and respect will be my highest priority—both with my partner and myself.

*Love and you shall be loved.*
*—Ralph Waldo Emerson*

# ACKNOWLEDGMENTS

Heartfelt thanks to my editor, Jodi Davis; illustrator, Thorina Rose;
publicist, Debbie Matsumoto; designer, Tim Belonax; managing
editors, Jan Hughes and Doug Ogan; copyeditor, Carolyn Miller.
**A special thanks to all my *Lovers' Yoga* stretching partners**.

# BIOGRAPHY

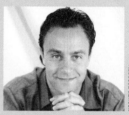

Rebecca Lawson

**Darrin Zeer** teaches Lovers' Yoga retreats
at spas and retreats around the world. He
also teaches Office Yoga to corporations
throughout America.

    Darrin spent seven years traveling
and studying yoga and meditation throughout Asia. He currently works as an author,
seminar leader, consultant, and spokesperson. He has appeared on
CNN, and in *Time* magazine, the *Wall Street Journal*, and the *New
York Times*. His focus is on helping people to have more peace and
joy in their lives. He currently lives in San Diego, California. Darrin
is also the author of *Office Yoga, Office Spa, Everyday Calm, Office
Feng Shui, Travel Yoga,* and *Office Stress Emergency Kit* (all from
Chronicle Books).

**Thorina Rose** is an award-winning illustrator. Her whimsical draw-
ings have appeared in *Office Kama Sutra* (from Chronicle Books) and
numerous publications. She lives in San Francisco.

To contact Darrin about his
Lovers' Yoga retreats,
go to **www.loversyoga.com**

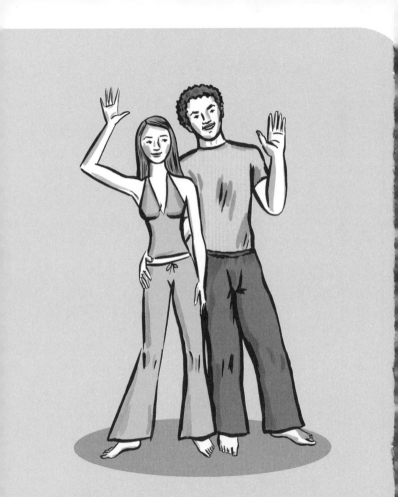

*There is nothing more important to each and every human being than love ... it is everything.*

—*Gourasana*